# Kettlebell Exercise Easy Guide for Beginners

## Intermediate Kettlebell Exercises

By

Lachlan Padraig

Copyright@2023

# Table of Contents

# CHAPTER 1

# Introduction

## 1.1 Why Kettlebell Exercises?

Kettlebell exercises have gained widespread popularity in the fitness world, and for good reason. They offer a unique and effective approach to strength training and overall fitness. Kettlebells are distinct from traditional dumbbells and barbells due to their compact, cannonball-like shape with a handle, which opens up a world of versatile exercises and training methods. So, why should you consider incorporating kettlebell exercises into your fitness routine?

Kettlebell exercises are a fantastic addition to your fitness repertoire for several compelling reasons. First and foremost, they provide a time-efficient and full-body workout that can help you achieve your fitness goals in a shorter amount of time. The unique design of the kettlebell allows for dynamic movements that engage multiple muscle groups simultaneously, promoting greater calorie expenditure and improved cardiovascular fitness. In other words, you can burn more calories and build strength simultaneously, making kettlebell exercises an excellent choice for those with busy schedules.

Additionally, kettlebell exercises offer a great way to develop functional strength. The movements involved in kettlebell training often mimic real-life activities and can enhance your ability to perform daily tasks with ease. This functional strength is not only beneficial for everyday life but also for various sports and athletic endeavors.

Another compelling reason to embrace kettlebell exercises is their versatility. They can be adapted to suit individuals of different fitness levels, from beginners to advanced athletes. Whether you're new to fitness or a seasoned pro, kettlebell exercises can be tailored to your specific needs and goals. This adaptability makes them an inclusive and accessible fitness tool.

## 1.2 Benefits of Kettlebell Training

Kettlebell training offers a multitude of benefits that extend far beyond just building muscle and increasing strength. Let's delve into some of the key advantages:

1. **Total Body Workout**: Kettlebell exercises engage multiple muscle groups simultaneously, providing a comprehensive full-body workout. This means you can work on your upper body, lower body, core, and even cardiovascular fitness in a single session.

2. **Functional Strength**: Kettlebell movements often mimic real-life activities, enhancing your functional

strength. This type of strength is crucial for maintaining independence and excelling in various physical pursuits.

3. **Improved Flexibility**: Kettlebell exercises require a wide range of motion, helping to improve flexibility and mobility. This can reduce the risk of injury and enhance your overall physical performance.

4. **Calorie Burning**: The dynamic nature of kettlebell exercises elevates your heart rate and burns a significant number of calories. This makes them an excellent choice for weight loss and fat loss goals.

5. **Enhanced Core Strength**: Many kettlebell exercises require a strong core for

stability and control. As a
result, you'll develop a robust
and functional core, which is
essential for good posture and
spine health.

6.  **Time Efficiency**: With
    kettlebell exercises, you can
    achieve a challenging workout
    in a relatively short amount of
    time. This is ideal for busy
    individuals looking to
    maximize the benefits of
    exercise within their time
    constraints.

7.  **Variety and Fun**: Kettlebell
    workouts can be engaging and
    enjoyable due to their variety.
    You can switch between
    different exercises and routines
    to keep your workouts
    interesting.

8. **Adaptability**: Kettlebell training can be tailored to suit different fitness levels and goals, whether you're a beginner, intermediate, or advanced athlete. The adaptability of kettlebells makes them a versatile training tool.

# 1.3 Safety Precautions

While kettlebell training offers numerous benefits, safety should always be a top priority to prevent injuries and ensure a positive training experience. Here are some essential safety precautions to keep in mind:

**Proper Form and Technique**: Before engaging in kettlebell exercises, it's crucial to learn and practice proper form and technique.

Using improper form can lead to injuries. Consider working with a certified kettlebell instructor or using instructional videos and resources to ensure you're performing exercises correctly.

**Start with the Right Weight**: Choose an appropriate kettlebell weight for your current fitness level. Beginning with a weight that is too heavy can lead to strain or injury. As a guideline, a beginner may start with an 8kg (18lbs) kettlebell for women and a 16kg (35lbs) kettlebell for men.

**Warm-Up and Cool Down**: Always incorporate warm-up and cool-down routines into your kettlebell workouts. Proper warm-up helps prepare your muscles and joints for exercise, while a cool-down aids in recovery and reduces muscle soreness.

**Listen to Your Body**: Pay attention to your body's signals during your workout. If you experience pain or discomfort, stop the exercise and seek guidance. Overexertion or pushing through pain can lead to injury.

**Progress Gradually**: Gradually increase the weight and intensity of your kettlebell exercises as you become more proficient. This allows your body to adapt safely and avoid overtraining.

**Stay Hydrated**: Adequate hydration is essential for any workout. Make sure to drink water before, during, and after your kettlebell training sessions.

**Consult a Physician**: If you have any underlying medical conditions or are new to exercise, consider consulting with a healthcare professional before starting a kettlebell training program.

kettlebell exercises offer a multitude of benefits, from total body workouts to enhanced functional strength and flexibility. By following safety precautions, practicing proper form, and progressively advancing your training, you can harness the power of kettlebells to achieve your fitness goals safely and effectively. Remember that consistency and patience are key to reaping the rewards of kettlebell training, and always prioritize your safety and well-being throughout your fitness journey.

# CHAPTER 2
# Getting Started

## 2.1 Choosing the Right Kettlebell

Selecting the appropriate kettlebell is the first step in your journey to effective kettlebell training. The right choice ensures that your workouts are safe, challenging, and align with your fitness goals. Here's what you need to consider when choosing a kettlebell:

- **Weight Selection**: Kettlebells come in various weights, typically ranging from 4kg (9lbs) to 48kg (106lbs) or more. As a beginner, start with a weight that allows you to perform exercises with proper form. For most women, an 8kg (18lbs) kettlebell is a good starting point, while men can begin with a 16kg (35lbs) kettlebell. However, these are general guidelines, and your fitness level, experience, and goals may necessitate a different starting weight.

- **Handle Diameter**: The handle's thickness and texture can vary among kettlebells. Choose a kettlebell with a handle diameter that fits comfortably in your hand and allows a secure grip. Ensure that it is not too thick or slippery, as this can lead to discomfort and poor control during exercises.

- **Quality**: Invest in high-quality kettlebells made of durable materials. Look for kettlebells with a smooth, even coating that won't cause friction against your skin or clothing. High-quality kettlebells are less likely to develop sharp edges that can cause injuries.

- **Single or Competition Style**: You'll encounter different styles of kettlebells, including traditional single-piece kettlebells and competition-style kettlebells with uniform dimensions regardless of weight. Your choice may depend on personal preference, training goals, and budget.

- **Consider Your Goals**: The weight of your kettlebell should align with your specific goals. Lighter kettlebells are suitable for high-repetition workouts and cardio, while heavier kettlebells are ideal for building strength and power. Think about your primary objectives when selecting a weight.

- **Space and Budget**: Determine the space you have available for your kettlebell workouts and your budget. If you have limited space, you may opt for a compact set of kettlebells that can be easily stored. Your budget will also influence the quality and variety of kettlebells you can acquire.

## 2.2 Proper Form and Technique

Mastering proper form and technique is the foundation of effective and safe

kettlebell training. Here's how to
ensure you're using the correct form:

- **Educate Yourself**: Before you
  start kettlebell training, educate
  yourself about the specific
  exercises you plan to perform.
  Seek guidance from certified
  instructors, watch instructional
  videos, and read books or
  articles on kettlebell
  techniques.

- **Start with the Basics**: Begin
  with fundamental kettlebell
  exercises like the two-handed
  swing and goblet squat. These
  exercises provide an excellent
  introduction to proper form and
  technique.

- **Maintain a Neutral Spine**:
  Keep your spine in a neutral
  position during kettlebell

exercises to avoid strain or injury. Engage your core muscles and maintain good posture throughout the movements.

- **Hinge at the Hips**: Many kettlebell exercises involve a hip hinge motion. This means bending at the hips while keeping your back straight, similar to a deadlift. The hinge is a fundamental movement pattern in kettlebell training.

- **Use Your Hips, Not Your Arms**: Kettlebell exercises rely on the power generated from your hips and core, not your arms. Avoid using your arms excessively; instead, focus on the hip drive to propel the kettlebell.

- **Practice Breathing**: Proper breathing is essential for maintaining stability and control during kettlebell exercises. Typically, you'll exhale forcefully during the exertion phase and inhale during the relaxation phase of an exercise.

- **Start with Light Weight**: When learning new exercises or refining your technique, start with a light kettlebell to minimize the risk of injury. Once you've mastered the form, gradually increase the weight.

- **Record and Review**: Consider recording yourself while performing kettlebell exercises. This allows you to review your form and make necessary adjustments.

- **Seek Feedback**: If possible, work with a certified kettlebell instructor who can provide personalized feedback and corrections.

## 2.3 Warm-Up and Stretching

Proper warm-up and stretching routines are crucial before engaging in kettlebell exercises. These preparatory activities help prevent injuries, improve performance, and enhance flexibility. Here are some guidelines for warming up and stretching:

- **General Warm-Up**: Start with a general warm-up, such as light jogging, jumping jacks, or dynamic movements that increase your heart rate and blood flow. Aim for 5-10 minutes of activity to raise your body temperature.

- **Joint Mobility Exercises**: Perform joint mobility exercises to loosen up and prepare your joints for movement. Focus on areas like the hips, shoulders, and spine.

- **Specific Warm-Up**: After your general warm-up, engage in a specific warm-up related to the exercises you plan to perform. For example, if you're doing kettlebell swings, start with a few sets of bodyweight swings to groove the movement pattern.

- **Dynamic Stretching**: Dynamic stretching involves moving your muscles and joints through a range of motion. Incorporate dynamic stretches like leg swings, arm circles, and hip rotations to further prepare your body.

- **Static Stretching**: After your workout, engage in static stretching to improve flexibility and reduce muscle tightness. Focus on the muscle groups you've worked during your kettlebell session.

- **Foam Rolling**: Consider using a foam roller to release muscle knots and tension. Foam rolling can be particularly beneficial for tight muscles before stretching.

- **Stay Hydrated**: Drink water before and during your warm-up to ensure proper hydration, which is essential for optimal muscle function.

A well-planned warm-up and stretching routine can help you perform kettlebell exercises with reduced risk of injury and enhanced physical performance. Never underestimate the importance of these preparatory activities in your kettlebell training journey.

# CHAPTER 3

# Basic Kettlebell Exercises

Incorporating basic kettlebell exercises into your fitness routine is an excellent way to build strength, improve your functional fitness, and boost your overall health. Here are five fundamental kettlebell exercises that form the foundation of many kettlebell workouts:

## 3.1 Two-Handed Kettlebell Swing

The two-handed kettlebell swing is a dynamic, full-body exercise that primarily targets the muscles of the posterior chain, including the glutes, hamstrings, and lower back. Here's how to perform the two-handed kettlebell swing:

**Step-by-Step:**

1.  Stand with your feet shoulder-width apart and place the kettlebell on the floor in front of you.

2.  Bend at your hips and knees to grasp the kettlebell handle with both hands, keeping your back straight and chest up.

3.  Swing the kettlebell backward between your legs, and then explosively thrust your hips forward to swing the kettlebell upward. The power should come from your hips, not your arms.

4. As the kettlebell reaches chest level, stand tall and engage your glutes and core.

5. Allow the kettlebell to swing back down between your legs and repeat the movement for your desired number of repetitions.

The two-handed kettlebell swing is an excellent exercise for building explosive hip power and cardiovascular endurance.

## 3.2 Single-Arm Kettlebell Swing

The single-arm kettlebell swing is a variation of the two-handed swing that emphasizes core and unilateral strength. It also engages your glutes, hamstrings, and lower back. Here's how to perform the single-arm kettlebell swing:

**Step-by-Step:**

1. Begin with your feet shoulder-width apart and the kettlebell on the floor in front of you.

2. Bend at your hips and knees to pick up the kettlebell with one hand, maintaining a straight back and an engaged core.

3. Swing the kettlebell backward between your legs and then powerfully thrust your hips forward to swing it upward.

4. At the top of the swing, the kettlebell should be at chest level. Maintain control and engage your core.

5. Allow the kettlebell to swing back down between your legs

and repeat the exercise for your desired number of repetitions.

6.  Switch hands and perform an equal number of repetitions on the other side.

The single-arm kettlebell swing helps improve balance and coordination while targeting one side of your body at a time, which can help address muscle imbalances.

## 3.3 Goblet Squat

The goblet squat is a powerful lower body exercise that not only builds strength in the quadriceps, hamstrings, and glutes but also engages your core and upper body. Here's how to perform the goblet squat:

**Step-by-Step:**

1.  Hold a kettlebell close to your chest with both hands, gripping the horns (the sides of the handle) or the base.

2.  Stand with your feet shoulder-width apart.

3.  Lower your body by bending at the hips and knees, keeping your chest up and back straight.

4.  Continue to squat until your thighs are parallel to the ground or as far as your flexibility allows.

5.  Push through your heels to stand back up and return to the starting position.

The goblet squat is an excellent exercise for developing leg strength, improving posture, and enhancing overall lower body function.

# 3.4 Kettlebell Deadlift

The kettlebell deadlift is a simple yet effective exercise for targeting the muscles of the lower back, glutes, and hamstrings. It also engages the core and upper body. Here's how to perform the kettlebell deadlift:

**Step-by-Step:**

1. Place a kettlebell on the ground in front of you.

2. Stand with your feet hip-width apart and your toes under the kettlebell.

3. Bend at your hips and knees to grasp the kettlebell handle with both hands.

4. Keep your back straight, chest up, and shoulders pulled back as you stand up, lifting the kettlebell with you.

5. Stand tall and engage your glutes at the top of the movement.

6. Lower the kettlebell back to the ground by bending at your hips and knees, maintaining proper form throughout.

The kettlebell deadlift is an excellent exercise for building lower back and hip strength, and it's particularly valuable for those new to weightlifting.

# 3.5 Kettlebell Turkish Get-Up

The kettlebell Turkish Get-Up is a complex, full-body exercise that enhances mobility, stability, and overall strength. It consists of several coordinated movements, making it essential to practice with proper form and technique. Here's how to perform the kettlebell Turkish Get-Up:

**Step-by-Step:**

1.  Start by lying on your back with a kettlebell in one hand, arm fully extended toward the ceiling.

2.  Bend your knee on the same side as the kettlebell and place your foot flat on the ground.

3.  Extend your free arm out to the side at a 45-degree angle.

4.  Keeping your eyes on the kettlebell, press the kettlebell up while simultaneously lifting your torso off the ground and shifting your weight onto your opposite elbow.

5. Push through your palm to raise your torso into a seated position, with your legs forming a 90-degree angle.

6. From here, bridge your hips off the ground, creating a straight line from your knees to your shoulder.

7. Sweep your extended leg under your body so that you're in a kneeling position.

8. Stand up, keeping the kettlebell locked out overhead.

9. Reverse the sequence to return to the starting position.

The kettlebell Turkish Get-Up is a multifaceted exercise that enhances strength, stability, and mobility, making it a valuable addition to your training routine as you progress in kettlebell training.

These basic kettlebell exercises provide a solid foundation for your kettlebell training journey, targeting different muscle groups and improving your overall fitness. Remember to focus on proper form and technique to maximize the benefits and reduce the risk of injury. As you become more proficient, you can incorporate these exercises into full-body workouts to achieve your fitness goals.

# CHAPTER 4

# Intermediate Kettlebell Exercises

Once you've mastered the basic kettlebell exercises, you can progress to intermediate exercises that offer new challenges and opportunities for strength and skill development. Here are five intermediate kettlebell exercises to take your training to the next level:

## 4.1 Kettlebell Clean and Press

The kettlebell clean and press is a compound exercise that combines two distinct movements: the clean and the press. It targets the entire upper body, including the shoulders, triceps, and back. Here's how to perform the kettlebell clean and press:

**Step-by-Step:**

1. Start with a kettlebell on the ground in front of you.

2. Stand with your feet shoulder-width apart.

3. Bend at your hips and knees to grasp the kettlebell handle with one hand.

4. Hike the kettlebell back between your legs.

5. Quickly extend your hips and stand up while pulling the kettlebell upward.

6. As the kettlebell rises, tuck your elbow to your side and

guide it to your shoulder in the clean motion.

7.  From the racked position, press the kettlebell overhead until your arm is fully extended.

8.  Lower the kettlebell back to the racked position.

9.  Finally, lower the kettlebell back to the ground with control.

The kettlebell clean and press is an excellent exercise for building strength, power, and coordination in the upper body.

## 4.2 Kettlebell Snatch

The kettlebell snatch is a dynamic, explosive movement that engages the entire body, with a focus on the shoulders, hips, and core. It involves lifting the kettlebell from the ground to an overhead position in a single fluid motion. Here's how to perform the kettlebell snatch:

**Step-by-Step:**

1.  Begin with a kettlebell on the ground in front of you.

2.  Stand with your feet shoulder-width apart.

3.  Bend at your hips and knees to grasp the kettlebell handle with one hand.

4.  Hike the kettlebell back between your legs.

5.  Explosively extend your hips and stand up while simultaneously pulling the kettlebell upward.

6. As the kettlebell rises, extend your arm fully overhead to finish in a locked-out position.

7. Lower the kettlebell back to the ground with control.

The kettlebell snatch is an advanced exercise that requires power, coordination, and proper technique. It's an efficient way to develop full-body strength and explosiveness.

# 4.3 Kettlebell Windmill

The kettlebell windmill is a mobility and stability exercise that targets the muscles of the core, shoulders, and hips. It also enhances flexibility. Here's how to perform the kettlebell windmill:

**Step-by-Step:**

1.  Stand with your feet wider than shoulder-width apart, with one kettlebell in one hand, arm extended overhead.

2.  Keep your feet pointing forward and the kettlebell arm on the same side as the working leg.

3.  While keeping your eyes on the kettlebell, hinge at your hips and bend laterally at the waist, lowering your opposite hand toward the ground.

4.  Maintain a straight arm and keep your chest open as you reach down.

5.  Once you've reached your comfortable range of motion, reverse the movement to return to the starting position.

6. Repeat for your desired number of repetitions.

The kettlebell windmill is an excellent exercise for improving shoulder mobility, core strength, and balance.

## 4.4 Kettlebell High Pull

The kettlebell high pull is a powerful exercise that targets the upper back, shoulders, and traps. It's an excellent movement for developing explosive strength. Here's how to perform the kettlebell high pull:

**Step-by-Step:**

1. Begin with a kettlebell on the ground between your feet.

2. Stand with your feet hip-width apart.

3.  Bend at your hips and knees to grasp the kettlebell handle with one hand.

4.  Hike the kettlebell back between your legs.

5.  Explosively extend your hips and stand up while pulling the kettlebell upward.

6.  As the kettlebell rises, bend your elbow to pull it up toward your shoulder, leading with your elbow.

7.  Lower the kettlebell back to the ground with control.

The kettlebell high pull is a dynamic exercise that enhances explosive power, shoulder strength, and upper back development.

# 4.5 Kettlebell Figure 8

The kettlebell figure 8 is a unique and challenging exercise that enhances hand-eye coordination, core stability, and overall body control. Here's how to perform the kettlebell figure 8:

**Step-by-Step:**

1. Stand with your feet shoulder-width apart, holding a kettlebell in one hand.

2. Begin by passing the kettlebell between your legs from the front to the back, moving it around one leg.

3. As the kettlebell comes around the opposite leg, reach through with the opposite hand to receive it.

4. Continue the figure-8 pattern between your legs, alternating

hands as the kettlebell goes
around each leg.

5. Maintain good posture and
control throughout the exercise.

The kettlebell figure 8 is a fun and functional exercise that enhances coordination and core strength, making it an excellent addition to your training routine.

These intermediate kettlebell exercises offer a higher level of complexity and challenge, helping you progress in your kettlebell training journey. Remember to prioritize proper form and technique to maximize the effectiveness of these exercises and reduce the risk of injury. As you become more proficient, you can incorporate these exercises into your workouts to continue improving your strength, power, and overall fitness.

# CHAPTER 5

# Advanced Kettlebell Exercises

Advanced kettlebell exercises offer a higher degree of difficulty and require enhanced strength, stability, and coordination. These movements can challenge even experienced individuals and are ideal for those looking to take their kettlebell training to the next level.

# 5.1 Kettlebell TGU (Turkish Get-Up) Variations

The Turkish Get-Up (TGU) is a complex, full-body exercise that involves a series of movements to transition from lying on your back to a standing position while holding a kettlebell overhead. There are various TGU variations that add complexity and challenge. Here's a general overview of the Turkish Get-Up:

**Step-by-Step for the Basic TGU:**

1.  Begin lying on your back with a kettlebell in one hand, arm extended toward the ceiling.

2.  Bend your knee on the same side as the kettlebell and place your foot flat on the ground.

3.  Keep your other leg extended, and your arm on the opposite side out to the side.

4.  Roll onto your side and use your free hand to push yourself into a seated position.

5.  From here, bridge your hips off the ground, creating a straight line from your knees to your shoulder.

6.  Sweep your extended leg under your body to come into a kneeling position.

7.  Stand up, keeping the kettlebell locked out overhead.

8.  Reverse the sequence to return to the starting position.

Turkish Get-Up variations can include holding the kettlebell in different positions, using a heavier kettlebell, or performing the TGU on an unstable surface.

## 5.2 Kettlebell Pistol Squat

The kettlebell pistol squat is a challenging single-leg squat that requires strength, balance, and flexibility. Here's how to perform the kettlebell pistol squat:

**Step-by-Step:**

1. Hold a kettlebell close to your chest with both hands.

2. Stand on one leg with the other leg extended in front of you.

3. Lower your body into a deep squat on the standing leg, while keeping the other leg elevated.

4.  Your goal is to reach a deep squat position with your thigh parallel to the ground.

5.  Push through your heel to stand back up.

6.  Repeat for your desired number of repetitions on one leg before switching to the other.

The kettlebell pistol squat is an advanced lower body exercise that targets the quadriceps, hamstrings, and glutes while enhancing balance and stability.

## 5.3 Kettlebell Renegade Rows

Kettlebell renegade rows are a challenging exercise that combines a push-up and a row, engaging the

chest, back, shoulders, and core.
Here's how to perform kettlebell
renegade rows:

**Step-by-Step:**

1.  Begin in a push-up position
    with one hand on a kettlebell
    and the other on the ground.

2.  Perform a push-up while
    maintaining a strong core and
    proper form.

3.  After completing the push-up,
    row the kettlebell to your hip,
    pulling your elbow high and
    engaging the lat.

4.  Lower the kettlebell back to the
    ground.

5.  Repeat the push-up and row on
    the other side.

6.  Continue alternating sides for your desired number of repetitions.

Kettlebell renegade rows are an excellent upper body exercise that enhances strength and core stability. They also challenge your coordination and balance.

These advanced kettlebell exercises provide a significant challenge to your strength, balance, and coordination. Ensure that you have mastered the basic and intermediate kettlebell exercises and have a solid foundation of strength and stability before attempting these advanced movements. It's essential to prioritize proper form and technique to perform these exercises safely and effectively. Advanced kettlebell exercises can offer a higher level of intensity and complexity, helping you achieve new fitness goals and continue progressing in your kettlebell training journey.

## 5.4 Kettlebell Juggling

Kettlebell juggling is an advanced and unconventional form of kettlebell training that involves dynamic and acrobatic movements with kettlebells. It combines strength, coordination, and agility in a unique way. Kettlebell juggling can include a wide range of movements, such as flips, spins, and catches, where the kettlebell is airborne. It's important to note that kettlebell juggling should only be attempted by experienced kettlebell enthusiasts, as it carries a higher risk of injury due to the dynamic and unpredictable nature of the exercises.

Kettlebell juggling offers a fun and creative way to challenge your skills, build strength, and improve hand-eye coordination. However, it's crucial to prioritize safety when engaging in these movements. Beginners or those new to kettlebell training should gain proficiency with fundamental kettlebell exercises and develop a solid foundation of strength and technique before attempting kettlebell juggling.

## 5.5 Kettlebell Complexes

Kettlebell complexes are a series of exercises performed consecutively without setting the kettlebell down. They are designed to provide a high-intensity full-body workout by combining different movements into a fluid sequence. Kettlebell complexes can be adapted for various fitness levels and goals, making them a versatile training method. Here's how to perform kettlebell complexes:

**Step-by-Step:**

1.  Choose a series of kettlebell exercises that flow well together, such as swings, cleans, presses, squats, or snatches.

2.  Perform each exercise in succession, one after the other, without resting or setting the kettlebell down.

3.  Once you've completed all the exercises in the complex, you can rest briefly before repeating the sequence for your desired number of rounds.

Kettlebell complexes are highly efficient and can be tailored to your fitness level and goals, whether you want to focus on building strength, improving cardiovascular fitness, or both. They provide a challenging workout that targets multiple muscle groups and can be a time-saving option for individuals with busy schedules. As with any kettlebell training, it's important to maintain proper form and technique to reduce the risk of injury while performing kettlebell complexes.

Both kettlebell juggling and kettlebell complexes offer advanced training options that can add variety and intensity to your workout routine. However, it's crucial to approach these advanced techniques with caution and consider seeking guidance from a qualified kettlebell instructor if you're not already experienced with these movements. Safety, proper form, and progressive training are key factors in successfully incorporating these advanced kettlebell exercises into your fitness regimen.

# CHAPTER 6

# Kettlebell Workout Routines

Kettlebell workouts are a fantastic way to improve your overall fitness and strength. Below is a beginner kettlebell workout routine that will help you get started on your journey to using this versatile piece of equipment effectively. This routine focuses on fundamental movements and is designed for beginners, but it can be adapted as your strength and experience increase.

# 6.1 Beginner Kettlebell Workout

**Warm-Up:**

- Perform 5-10 minutes of light cardiovascular activity to raise your heart rate and prepare your muscles for exercise. You can do jumping jacks, jogging in place, or even brisk walking.

**Workout:**

1. **Two-Handed Kettlebell Swing** - 3 sets of 12-15 reps

   - Stand with your feet shoulder-width apart.

   - Hold the kettlebell with both hands, keeping your arms extended.

   - Bend at your hips and knees, swinging the

kettlebell back between
your legs.

- Explosively thrust your
  hips forward to swing the
  kettlebell to chest level.

- Repeat the swing for the
  prescribed number of
  reps.

2. **Goblet Squat** - 3 sets of 10-12
reps

- Hold the kettlebell close
  to your chest with both
  hands.

- Stand with your feet
  shoulder-width apart.

- Lower your body into a
  squat, keeping your back
  straight and chest up.

- Push through your heels
  to stand back up.

3. **Kettlebell Deadlift** - 3 sets of
   10-12 reps

   - Place the kettlebell on
     the ground in front of
     you.

   - Stand with your feet hip-
     width apart.

   - Bend at your hips and
     knees to grasp the
     kettlebell handle with
     both hands.

   - Keep your back straight
     as you stand up, lifting
     the kettlebell with you.

   - Lower the kettlebell back
     to the ground with
     control.

4.  **Kettlebell Turkish Get-Up
    (Partial)** - 3 sets of 2-3 reps per
    side

    - Lie on your back with a
      kettlebell in one hand,
      arm extended toward the
      ceiling.

    - Follow the steps of the
      Turkish Get-Up until you
      reach the seated position,
      then reverse the
      movement.

    - Repeat for the prescribed
      number of reps on each
      side.

**Cool Down:**

- Finish your workout with 5-10
  minutes of stretching to
  improve flexibility and reduce
  muscle soreness. Focus on

stretches for the muscles worked during the workout, such as the hips, hamstrings, and shoulders.

**Notes:**

- Start with a light to moderate weight kettlebell that allows you to perform each exercise with proper form.

- Rest for 1-2 minutes between sets.

- Focus on using proper form and technique throughout the workout to avoid injury.

- As you become more comfortable with the exercises, you can gradually increase the weight of your kettlebell or add more sets and repetitions to challenge yourself.

This beginner kettlebell workout routine provides a well-rounded introduction to kettlebell training. It targets major muscle groups while also working on coordination and balance. As you progress, you can modify and expand your routines to include more advanced kettlebell exercises and training methods. Always prioritize safety and proper technique in your workouts.

## 6.2 Intermediate Kettlebell Workout

If you have mastered the basics of kettlebell training and want to take your workouts to the next level, this intermediate kettlebell workout is designed to challenge your strength, endurance, and coordination. This routine includes a mix of intermediate exercises to provide a comprehensive full-body workout.

## Warm-Up:

- Start with 5-10 minutes of light cardio to get your heart rate up and prepare your body for exercise.

## Workout:

1. **Kettlebell Clean and Press** - 3 sets of 8-10 reps per arm

    - Clean the kettlebell from the ground to the racked position.

    - Press it overhead, fully extending your arm.

    - Lower the kettlebell back to the ground and repeat for the prescribed number of reps on each arm.

2. **Kettlebell Snatch** - 3 sets of 10-12 reps per arm

  - Perform snatches with one arm at a time.

  - Swing the kettlebell between your legs and explosively bring it overhead.

  - Lower it back to the ground and switch arms for each set.

3. **Kettlebell Goblet Squat** - 3 sets of 12-15 reps

  - Hold a kettlebell close to your chest with both hands.

- Perform deep squats with proper form and control.

4. **Kettlebell High Pull** - 3 sets of 10-12 reps per arm

   - Hike the kettlebell back between your legs.

   - Swing it upward and pull it toward your shoulder.

   - Alternate arms for each set.

5. **Kettlebell Windmill** - 3 sets of 8-10 reps per side

   - Hold the kettlebell overhead with one arm.

   - Bend laterally at the waist while keeping your eyes on the kettlebell.

- Perform the windmill for the prescribed number of reps on each side.

**Cool Down:**

- Finish with 5-10 minutes of stretching to improve flexibility and reduce muscle tension. Focus on stretching the major muscle groups worked during the workout.

**Notes:**

- Use a kettlebell weight that challenges you but allows you to maintain proper form.

- Rest for 1-2 minutes between sets.

- Ensure that you use proper technique for each exercise to minimize the risk of injury.

- As you progress, you can increase the weight of your kettlebell, add more sets or repetitions, or decrease rest periods to intensify your workouts.

This intermediate kettlebell workout incorporates more complex movements and a higher level of intensity to build on the foundation of your kettlebell training. Always prioritize safety, technique, and progressive overload in your workouts. As you continue to advance, you can explore advanced kettlebell exercises and training methods to further enhance your fitness and strength.

# 6.3 Advanced Kettlebell Workout

An advanced kettlebell workout is designed for individuals who have a strong foundation in kettlebell training and are looking to push their limits further. This workout incorporates challenging exercises to improve strength, endurance, and overall fitness. Here's an advanced kettlebell workout:

**Warm-Up:**

- Perform a 10-minute dynamic warm-up to increase blood flow and mobility. Include exercises like leg swings, arm circles, and bodyweight squats.

**Workout:**

1. **Kettlebell Clean and Press** - 4 sets of 6-8 reps per arm

- Clean the kettlebell to the racked position.

- Press it overhead with a full lockout.

- Lower the kettlebell back to the ground and switch arms for each set.

2. **Kettlebell Snatch** - 4 sets of 10-12 reps per arm

- Perform snatches with one arm at a time.

- Focus on a smooth, powerful motion.

- Switch arms for each set.

3. **Kettlebell Pistol Squat** - 4 sets of 6-8 reps per leg

- Perform pistol squats, one-legged squats, with proper form.

- Use a kettlebell for balance and counterbalance as needed.

4. **Kettlebell Renegade Rows** - 4 sets of 8-10 reps per arm

   - Get into a push-up position with a kettlebell in each hand.

   - Perform a push-up and row one kettlebell, then switch to the other side for each rep.

5. **Kettlebell Turkish Get-Up (Full)** - 3 sets of 2-3 reps per arm

   - Execute the full Turkish Get-Up, starting from a lying position and ending in a standing position.

- Complete the prescribed number of reps on each arm.

**Cool Down:**

- Spend 10-15 minutes on static stretching to improve flexibility and reduce muscle tension. Focus on the major muscle groups worked during the workout.

**Notes:**

- Select a challenging kettlebell weight, but one that allows you to maintain proper form.

- Rest for 1-2 minutes between sets.

- Focus on maintaining perfect technique throughout the workout to minimize the risk of injury.

- As you progress, you can increase the weight, add more sets or reps, or reduce rest periods to intensify your workouts.

This advanced kettlebell workout is designed to challenge your strength, balance, and overall fitness. Ensure you have a solid foundation in kettlebell training before attempting these advanced exercises. Always prioritize safety, form, and proper technique in your workouts.

## 6.4 Kettlebell HIIT (High-Intensity Interval Training)

Kettlebell HIIT is a high-intensity interval training workout that combines kettlebell exercises with cardiovascular elements for a full-body, calorie-burning workout. HIIT is a great way to improve cardiovascular fitness, burn fat, and build strength simultaneously. Here's a sample kettlebell HIIT workout:

**Warm-Up:**

- Perform 5-10 minutes of light cardio to get your heart rate up and prepare your body for exercise.

**Workout:**

Perform each exercise for 40 seconds, followed by a 20-second rest, and then move on to the next exercise. Complete the circuit for a total of 3-4 rounds:

1. **Kettlebell Swing** - Swing the kettlebell with proper form and control.

2.  **Kettlebell Goblet Squat** -
    Hold the kettlebell close to
    your chest and perform deep
    squats.

3.  **Kettlebell Clean and Press** -
    Clean the kettlebell and press it
    overhead.

4.  **Kettlebell Renegade Rows** -
    Get into a push-up position
    with a kettlebell in each hand,
    perform a push-up, and row one
    kettlebell.

**Cool Down:**

- Finish with 5-10 minutes of
  stretching to improve flexibility
  and reduce muscle tension.
  Focus on the major muscle
  groups worked during the
  workout.

**Notes:**

- Choose a kettlebell weight that challenges you without compromising form.

- Rest for 1-2 minutes between rounds.

- Focus on proper form and technique to minimize the risk of injury.

- Kettlebell HIIT workouts are intense, so ensure you're adequately conditioned before attempting them.

Kettlebell HIIT workouts are an effective way to boost your fitness level, shed unwanted pounds, and improve your strength. They can be tailored to your fitness level and goals. Always prioritize safety and proper form when incorporating HIIT workouts into your training routine.

# CHAPTER 7

# Tips for Success

## 7.1 Setting Goals

Setting clear and achievable goals is essential for success in kettlebell training, just as it is in any fitness endeavor. Here are some tips for setting and achieving your kettlebell training goals:

1. **Specificity**: Define your goals with clarity. Instead of saying, "I want to get better at kettlebell training," specify what you want to achieve, such as "I want to increase my kettlebell swing weight by 10 pounds in three months."

2. **Realistic Goals**: Ensure your goals are achievable and realistic for your current fitness level. Setting overly ambitious goals can lead to frustration and potential injury. Gradual progress is sustainable progress.

3. **Short-Term and Long-Term Goals**: Set both short-term and long-term goals. Short-term goals can help you stay motivated and measure your progress along the way to your more significant, long-term objectives.

4. **S.M.A.R.T. Goals**: Use the S.M.A.R.T. criteria for goal setting:

- **S**pecific: Make your goals specific and precise.

- **M**easurable: Ensure you can measure your progress.

- **A**ttainable: Make sure your goals are achievable.

- **R**elevant: Ensure your goals align with your overall objectives.

- **T**ime-bound: Set a deadline for achieving your goals.

5. **Adaptability**: Be open to adjusting your goals as you progress. Sometimes you may realize that a different path or

outcome is more appropriate as you gain experience.

6. **Consistency**: Consistently working towards your goals is key. Develop a routine and stick to it, as consistency is crucial for success.

7. **Celebrate Milestones**: Celebrate your achievements along the way. Recognizing your progress, no matter how small, can boost motivation and help you stay on track.

8. **Stay Accountable**: Share your goals with a friend or trainer, or use a training journal to track your progress. Being accountable to someone or something can help keep you focused.

# 7.2 Progress Tracking

Tracking your progress is essential to monitor your improvements, identify areas for refinement, and stay motivated. Here are some tips for effective progress tracking in kettlebell training:

1. **Training Journal**: Keep a training journal where you record your workouts, including exercises, sets, reps, weights, and any notes about your performance. This allows you to see how you're progressing over time.

2. **Measurements and Photos**: Take measurements of your body (e.g., waist, hips, and chest) and periodic photos to visually track changes in your physique and muscle definition.

3.  **Strength and Endurance
    Testing**: Regularly assess your
    strength and endurance by
    testing your one-repetition
    maximum (1RM) for specific
    exercises or tracking how many
    repetitions you can perform
    with a given weight.

4.  **Performance Metrics**: Pay
    attention to performance
    metrics such as your time or
    distance in kettlebell swings,
    snatches, or other exercises.
    Monitor your ability to
    complete more repetitions or
    reduce the time taken for
    specific workouts.

5.  **Fitness Apps and Devices**:
    Consider using fitness apps,
    smartwatches, or other devices
    to track your workouts, heart
    rate, and progress. Many of

these tools provide insights and data on your fitness journey.

6. **Periodic Assessments**: Schedule regular assessments or check-ins with a fitness professional to evaluate your progress, receive feedback, and adjust your training plan as needed.

7. **Set Benchmarks**: Establish benchmark workouts or exercises that you revisit regularly to gauge your progress and make comparisons.

8. **Nutritional Tracking**: Remember that nutrition plays a significant role in your progress. Monitor your diet and adjust it as necessary to support your training goals.

9.  **Mindfulness**: Pay attention to how you feel physically, emotionally, and mentally during your workouts. Improved mood, reduced stress, and better sleep can be positive indicators of progress.

10. **Stay Patient**: Progress may not always be linear, and plateaus can occur. Be patient, stay committed, and trust the process.

By setting clear goals and consistently tracking your progress, you can make the most of your kettlebell training and stay motivated throughout your fitness journey. Celebrate your successes, learn from your challenges, and continue to refine your approach as you work towards your objectives.

# 7.3 Nutrition and Recovery

Proper nutrition and recovery are vital components of a successful kettlebell training program. They support your performance, muscle growth, and overall health. Here are some tips for nutrition and recovery in kettlebell training:

**Nutrition:**

1. **Balanced Diet**: Consume a well-balanced diet that includes a variety of whole foods, including lean protein, complex carbohydrates, healthy fats, and plenty of fruits and vegetables.

2. **Adequate Protein**: Protein is essential for muscle repair and growth. Ensure you get enough lean protein sources in your

diet, such as chicken, turkey, fish, tofu, and beans.

3. **Hydration**: Stay well-hydrated. Dehydration can impair your performance and hinder recovery.

4. **Pre-Workout Nutrition**: Fuel your body with a light, balanced meal or snack before your workout, including carbohydrates for energy.

5. **Post-Workout Nutrition**: After your workout, consume a combination of protein and carbohydrates to aid recovery and muscle repair. This can be in the form of a protein shake or a balanced meal.

6. **Healthy Snacking**: Choose nutritious snacks like nuts, yogurt, or fruit to maintain

energy levels throughout the day.

7. **Supplements**: Consider supplements like protein powder, creatine, and branched-chain amino acids (BCAAs) to support muscle growth and recovery, but consult with a healthcare professional before using them.

**Recovery:**

8. **Sleep**: Prioritize sleep. Your body repairs and rebuilds during sleep, so aim for 7-9 hours of quality sleep each night.

9. **Rest Days**: Incorporate rest days into your training program. Your body needs time to recover to prevent

overtraining and reduce the risk
of injury.

10. **Active Recovery**: On rest days,
    engage in light, low-impact
    activities like walking or yoga
    to maintain blood flow and
    flexibility.

11. **Foam Rolling and Stretching**:
    Use foam rolling and stretching
    to relieve muscle tension and
    improve flexibility.

12. **Hydration**: Stay hydrated
    throughout the day, as
    dehydration can lead to muscle
    cramps and delayed recovery.

13. **Nutrient Timing**: Consider the
    timing of your meals. Eating a
    balanced meal within 2 hours
    after your workout can aid
    recovery.

# 7.4 Common Mistakes to Avoid

Avoiding common mistakes in kettlebell training is crucial to prevent injury, maximize results, and stay on track with your fitness goals. Here are some common mistakes to be aware of:

1. **Poor Form**: Using improper form during exercises can lead to injury. Take the time to learn and practice proper form for each kettlebell exercise.

2. **Starting Too Heavy**: Beginning with a kettlebell that is too heavy can hinder your progress and increase the risk of injury. Start with a weight that allows you to perform exercises with good form.

3. **Neglecting Warm-Up and Cool-Down**: Skipping warm-up and cool-down routines can lead to muscle strains and reduced flexibility. Always incorporate these into your workouts.

4. **Overtraining**: Overtraining can lead to burnout, fatigue, and increased injury risk. Allow your body adequate rest and recovery time between workouts.

5. **Ignoring Nutrition**: Nutrition is a significant part of training success. Neglecting a balanced diet can hinder your progress and energy levels.

6. **Neglecting Mobility Work**: Flexibility and mobility are essential for kettlebell training.

Don't overlook stretching and mobility exercises.

7. **Not Progressing Safely**: While it's essential to challenge yourself, progressing too quickly in weight or intensity can lead to injury. Gradually increase the weight or intensity as your strength improves.

8. **Lack of Variety**: Doing the same exercises repeatedly can lead to plateaus and boredom. Include a variety of exercises in your routine to keep things interesting and challenge different muscle groups.

9. **Not Listening to Your Body**: Ignoring pain or discomfort can lead to injury. If something doesn't feel right, modify your

routine or seek guidance from a professional.

10. **Skipping Recovery Days**: Failing to include rest and recovery days in your training program can lead to overuse injuries. Make rest a priority.

Avoiding these common mistakes and paying attention to your form, nutrition, and recovery, you can have a more successful and sustainable kettlebell training experience. Always prioritize safety and take a holistic approach to your fitness journey.

## 7.5 Embracing a Kettlebell Training Lifestyle

Embracing a kettlebell training lifestyle means making kettlebell workouts and related fitness activities a consistent and integral part of your daily life. It's about incorporating fitness, nutrition, and overall wellness into your routine to achieve a healthy and active lifestyle. Here are some tips to help you embrace a kettlebell training lifestyle:

1. **Consistency**: Make kettlebell training a regular part of your routine. Aim for a minimum number of workouts each week, and be consistent with your training schedule.

2. **Set Goals**: Continuously set and work towards fitness goals

related to kettlebell training. Having goals keeps you motivated and focused.

3. **Holistic Health**: Understand that kettlebell training is just one component of a healthy lifestyle. Focus on overall wellness, including nutrition, sleep, stress management, and mental well-being.

4. **Nutrition**: Pay attention to your diet. Consume a balanced and nutritious diet that supports your fitness goals. Remember that what you eat plays a significant role in your overall health and performance.

5. **Recovery**: Prioritize recovery. Give your body the time it needs to repair and regenerate by getting enough sleep,

incorporating rest days, and engaging in active recovery.

6. **Learn Continuously**: Keep learning and expanding your knowledge about kettlebell training and related fitness concepts. Staying informed helps you make informed decisions about your training and health.

7. **Variety**: Embrace variety in your training. Include different kettlebell exercises and workouts to keep things interesting and challenge your body in new ways.

8. **Active Lifestyle**: Look for opportunities to stay active throughout the day, even when you're not working out. Walk more, take the stairs, and

engage in physical activities
you enjoy.

9.  **Mindset**: Cultivate a positive
    and growth-oriented mindset.
    Stay motivated, overcome
    challenges, and believe in your
    ability to achieve your fitness
    goals.

10. **Community**: Connect with
    others who share your passion
    for kettlebell training. Join
    fitness classes, find training
    partners, or engage with online
    communities to stay motivated
    and learn from others.

11. **Listen to Your Body**: Pay
    attention to your body's signals.
    If you're tired or not feeling
    your best, it's okay to adjust
    your training or take a break.

12. **Consistent Progress**: Aim for gradual and consistent progress over time. Don't expect instant results, and be patient with your fitness journey.

13. **Balance**: Strive for a balance between your fitness goals and other life priorities. A well-rounded life includes time for family, work, hobbies, and relaxation.

14. **Stay Inspired**: Find inspiration from fitness influencers, role models, and success stories in the kettlebell training community. Surround yourself with positive influences.

15. **Celebrate Achievements**: Celebrate your achievements, no matter how small they may seem. Each step towards your

goals is a reason to be proud of yourself.

Embracing a kettlebell training lifestyle is about making fitness a sustainable and enjoyable part of your life. It's not a short-term endeavor but a long-term commitment to your health and well-being. By following these tips and staying dedicated to your training, you can create a lifestyle that supports your fitness goals and contributes to your overall happiness and health.